Dear Mackenzie and Olivia,

Life is good

Enjoy Yoga

Cheers,

10/16/2012.

Dedicated to my students and
my granddaughter, Shreeya.
Pooja, you are my inspiration.

A big "thank you" to my
Yoga-loving family. I couldn't
have done it without your
love and support.

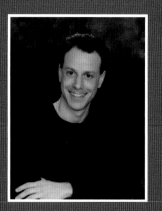

A sleepy cat wakes up from an afternoon nap and stretches out her limbs, arching her back, and then pressing down front paws onto the ground, in what we recognize as Yoga like poses. A bird stretches her wings just before taking off into the air. We, as children and adults, also stretch our bodies and strengthen our muscles in the Yoga movements that have been named after the familiar movements of animals, such as the cat pose or the dog pose. We do Yoga for the benefit of the stretch, but we also enjoy it for the lightness of our mind and to kindle our playful spirit.

We like to jump, extend our arms and see how far our legs can reach into the air, twist our bodies around, and find a moment of quiet when we lie down for our meditation at the end of our Yoga practice. Try doing Yoga if you want a new physical adventure and want to understand why all the animals we know stretch their limbs. In the end, we are all part of the same family of living creatures on this planet that enjoy movement, playfulness, and friendship.

David Rosenberg

PRT0412A

Printed in the United States

Library of Congress Control Number: 2012933176

ISBN-13: 978-1-937406-75-2
ISBN-10: 1-937406-75-X

www.mascotbooks.com

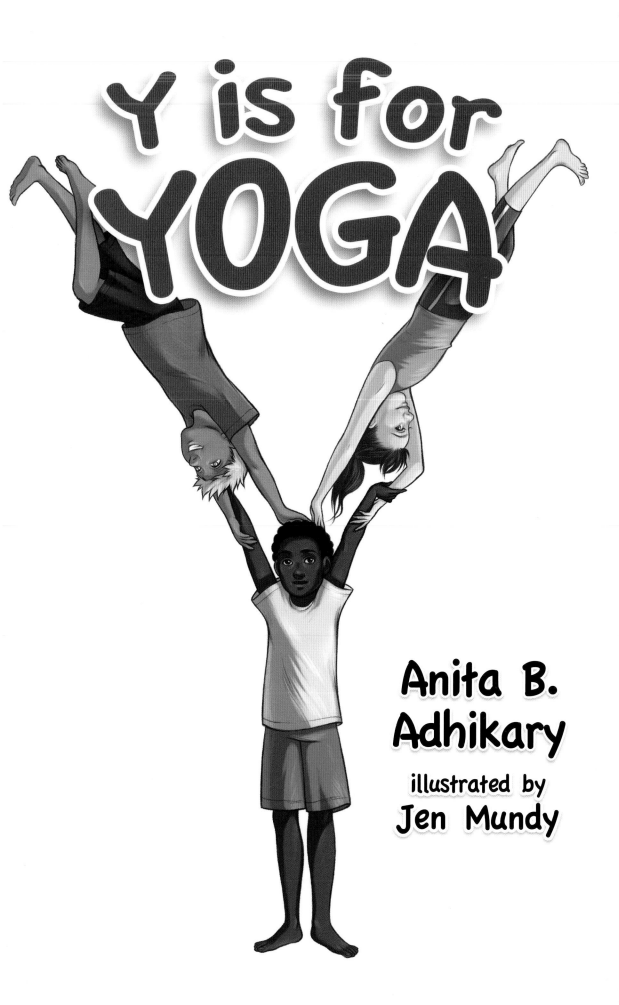

Y is for YOGA

Anita B. Adhikary

illustrated by
Jen Mundy

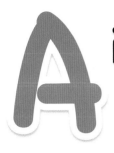 is for Attention

The essence of Yoga is attention and focus. It is important to pay attention to what you are doing and how you are breathing. You concentrate better when you breathe properly, and concentration helps you balance your poses much better.

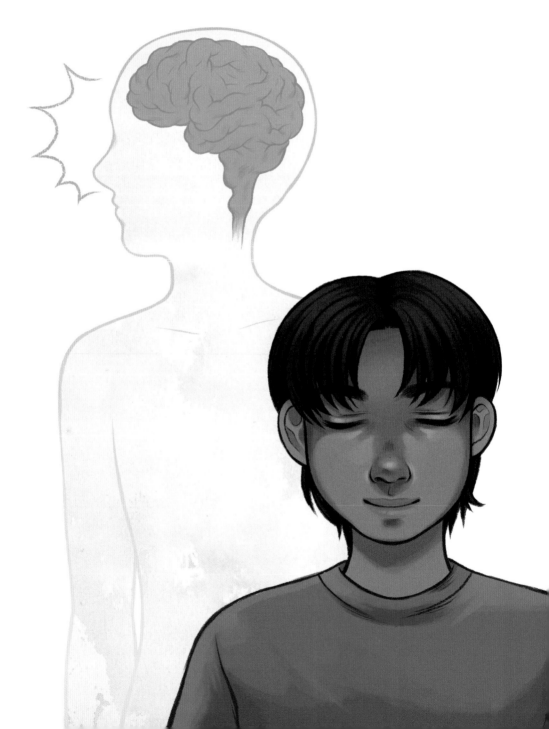

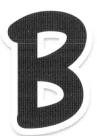

B is for Butterfly Pose

1. Inhale and sit down with a straight back. Exhale and stretch your legs out.
2. Inhale while slowly and steadily bringing your feet close to your pelvic area.
3. Exhale until the soles of your feet are touching each other.
4. Stretch your hands forward and reach down to hold your ankles.
4. Inhale and slowly lift your legs up. Try to flap your legs like wings.
5. Exhale and keep flapping your butterfly wings.
(Can you make butterfly antennas with your fingers?)

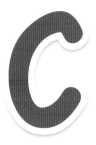

C is for Cobra Pose

1. Lie on your stomach with your legs and feet close together, and your palms on the mat next to your shoulders.

2. Inhale and lift your torso by straightening your arms. Try to lift your torso as far from the mat as possible. You now look like a cobra!

(Can you stick your tongue out and make a hissing sound like a snake?)

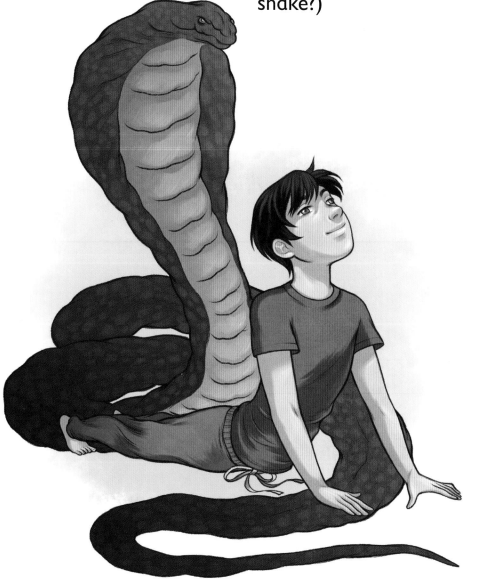

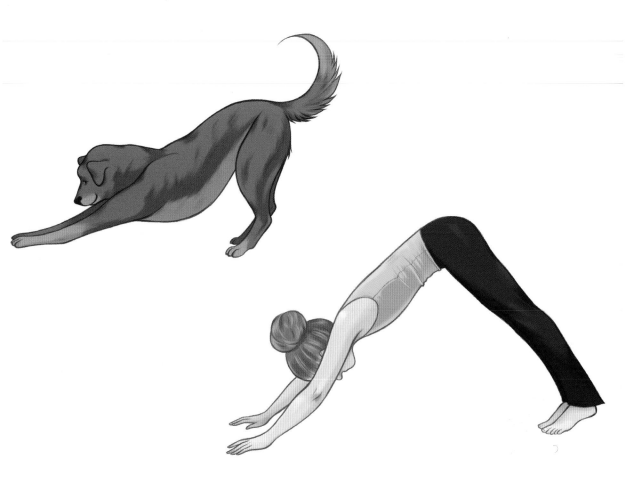

D is for Downward Facing Dog Pose

Have you ever noticed how a dog stretches after waking up? This pose is just like that!

1. Inhale and get down on your hands and knees.
2. Spread your fingers wide and push your hands forward on the mat.
3. Exhale and drop your head down until your ears are between your arms.
4. Slowly straighten your legs and sink your shoulders into the mat.

(Can you bark like a dog or wag your tail?)

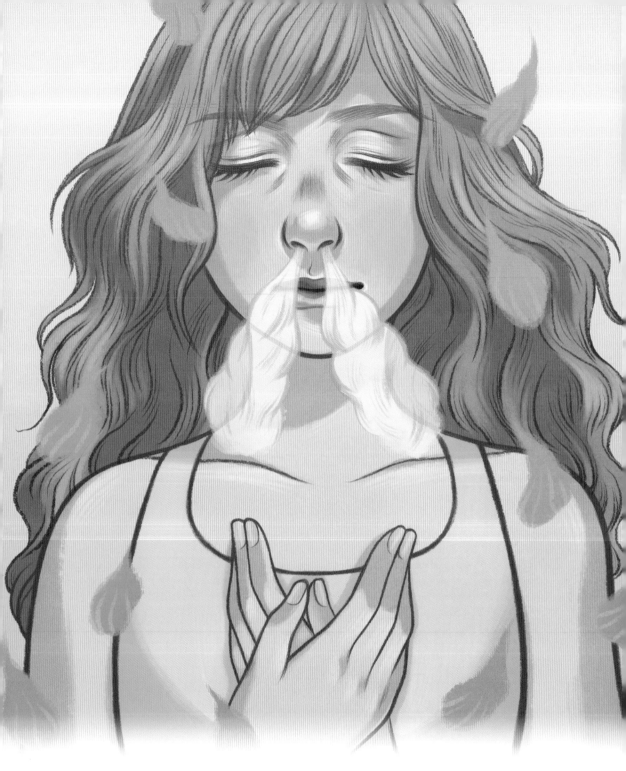

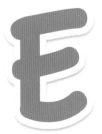 **is for Exhale**

Exhale means to breathe out carbon dioxide.
In Yoga, it is very important to exhale
properly through your nostrils.
(Do you know where we get our oxygen from?)

F is for Frog Pose

1. Inhale and stand tall and straight.
2. Exhale and squat down on your feet.
3. Inhale while bringing your legs together and leap like a frog.

(Can you make frog sounds?)

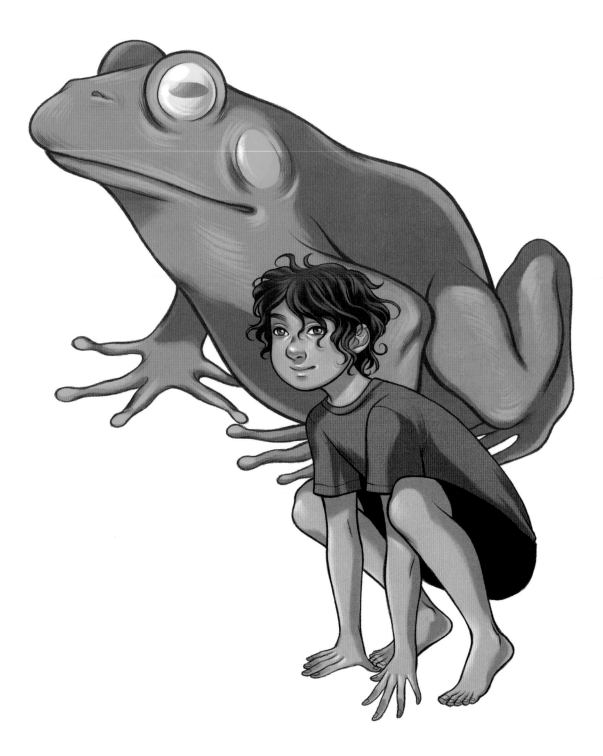

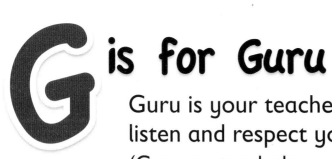

G is for Guru

Guru is your teacher. It is important to listen and respect your teacher.
(Can you teach the word *guru* to someone?)

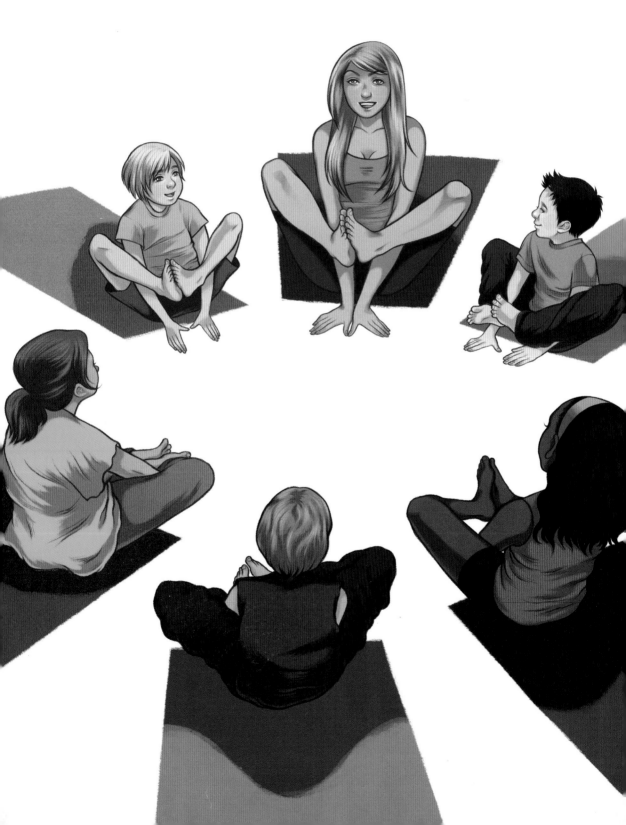

H is for Hand to Feet Pose

1. Stand straight and tall.
2. Inhale and raise your arms above your head.
3. Exhale and slowly bend forward to touch your feet.
4. Inhale and grasp your toes.

(Can you touch your toes yet? Keep practicing, and soon you will.)

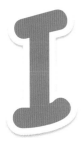

I is for Inhale

Inhale means breathing in oxygen. Breath is the fuel of life. The way you breathe is very important for practicing Yoga. Deep breathing, like what we do in Yoga, allows oxygen to travel to different parts of your body effectively helping your body function better.

(Do you know how oxygen travels all around your body?)

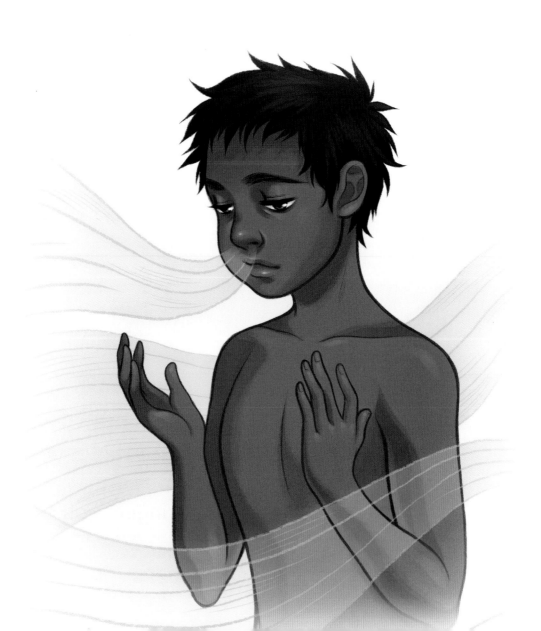

J is for Jump

1. Inhale and jump while spreading your arms and legs as wide as you can.
2. Exhale and jump while bringing your arms and legs back together.

(Can you do five sets of five jumping jacks?)

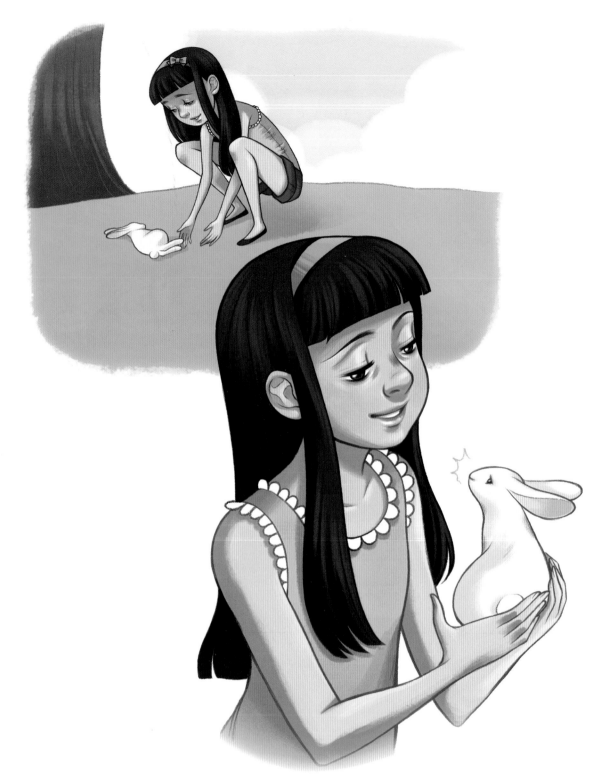

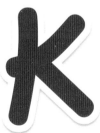 **is for Kindness**

We should be kind and take good care of our bodies. We can do this by eating healthy, becoming active, and remaining peaceful. (Have you done something kind today?)

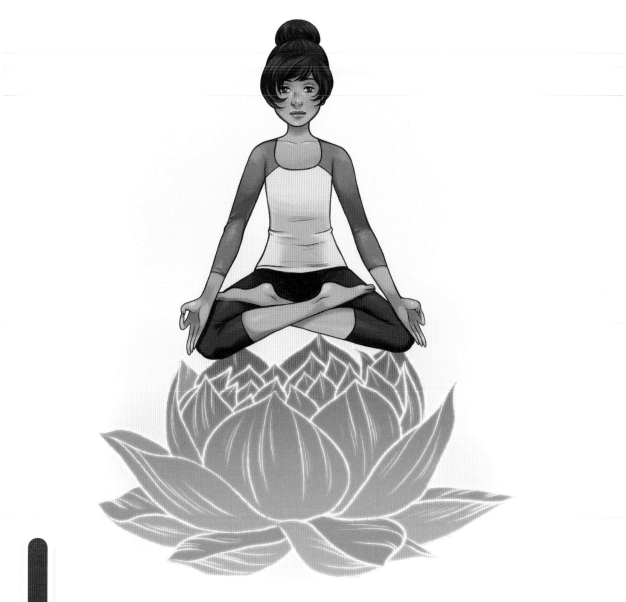

L is for Lotus Pose

Lotus is the most important pose in Yoga. This pose helps you meditate. You need to be comfortable, relaxed, and alert in this pose.

1. Sit with your legs crossed and your spine straight.
2. Fix your gaze on a focal point.
3. Stretch both your hands and bring them down to rest on your knees, palms up.
4. Join your thumb and your index finger on both hands.
5. Focus on deep breathing.

(Can you teach this pose to someone and help them meditate?)

M is for Mountain Pose

1. Stand with your feet together and your hands at your sides.
2. Hold this pose for five full breaths. Be sure to practice deep breathing.
(Can you stand still and majestic, just like Mount Everest?)

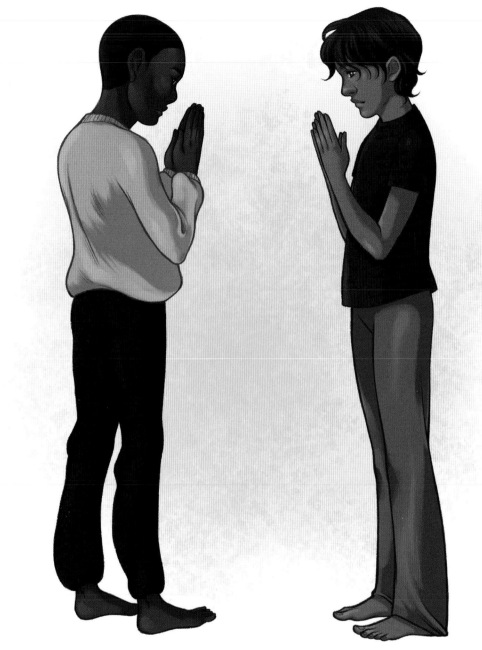

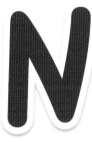 **is for Namaskar or Namaste**

Put your palms together and say, "Namaskar." This means you are greeting someone from within your soul.

(Can you say *namaskar* to your guru at the beginning of Yoga?)

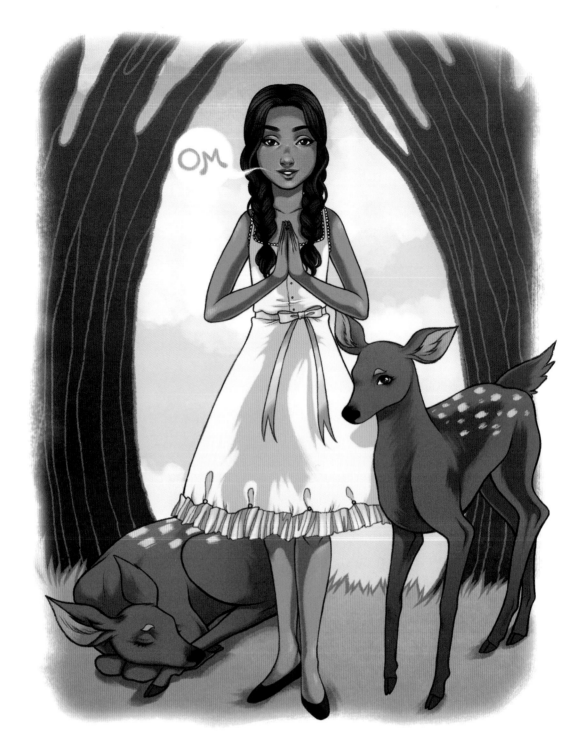

 **is for Om**

After you finish practicing Yoga, bring your palms together and say, "Om," to honor yourself and nature.

(Can you say *Om* at the end of Yoga?)

 # P is for Props

Some Yoga poses call for certain props or accessories. The props we use in Yoga are belts, blocks, mats, blankets, and water bottles.

(Do you know the shapes of these props? Are they rectangles? Are they cubes?)

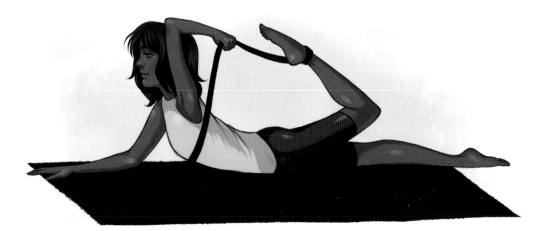

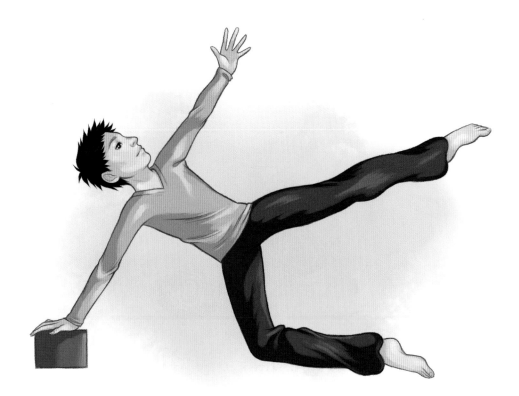

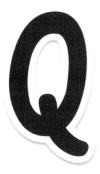is for Quiet

Remain quiet during Yoga practice. Sit quietly, be relaxed and calm. This helps with your concentration and focus. Your mind and body feel connected and you become peaceful.

(Do you know the Silence Game? The Silence Game can be played anywhere. Everybody sits in a circle, closes their eyes, and tries to remain very quiet, until the leader tells them to open their eyes. The leader asks them what sounds they heard. You will be amazed at what you hear when you are very quiet.)

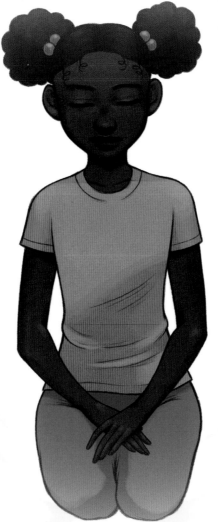

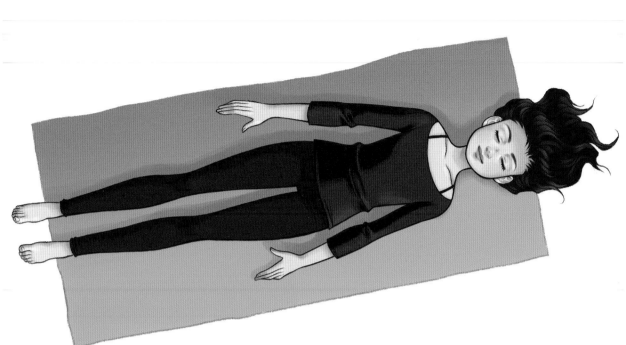

R is for Relaxation Pose

Relaxation is the pose that we practice last.
1. Lie on your back, close your eyes, and let your hands fall to your sides.
2. Start at your toes and imagine you are saying to them, "Relax toes." At the same time, take a deep breath, hold it for three seconds, and then exhale. Do this deep breathing with each body part.
3. Move up the rest of your body. Relax your ankles, shins, knees, and so on. Be sure to practice deep breathing at each body part.
4. Slowly sit up in a lotus pose and open your eyes.
(Can you concentrate on being quiet and breathing at the same time? You must be proud of yourself!)

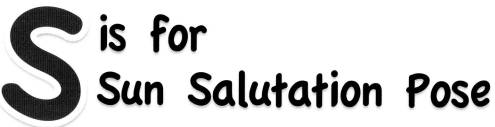

S is for Sun Salutation Pose

A great way to start the day is by greeting the sun.

(Can you do all of these poses one at a time?)

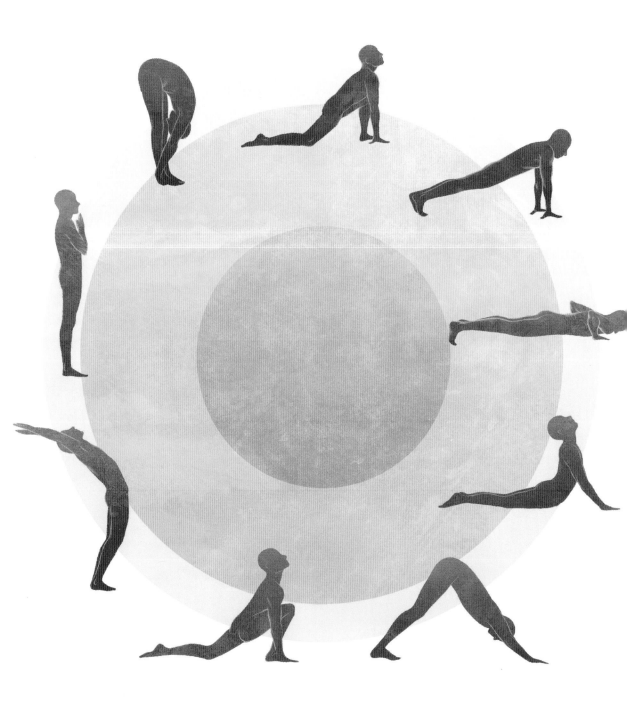

T is for Tree Pose

Think of a beautiful, strong, and old tree. Now try to become that tree.

1. Inhale and stand tall and straight.
2. Exhale and gently place your left foot on the inside of your right leg.
3. Inhale and stretch your arms sideways, as if they are branches.
4. Exhale and bring your palms together.
5. Raise your hands high above your head, keeping your palms together. You might lose your balance at first, but with practice you will become strong and steady like a tree.

(Can you stand for the full thirty seconds? Don't worry, you'll get there! Keep practicing!)

U is for Understanding Yourself

You know your body best. While practicing Yoga, be mindful and avoid doing poses that could hurt you. If you feel any discomfort or pain, immediately stop!

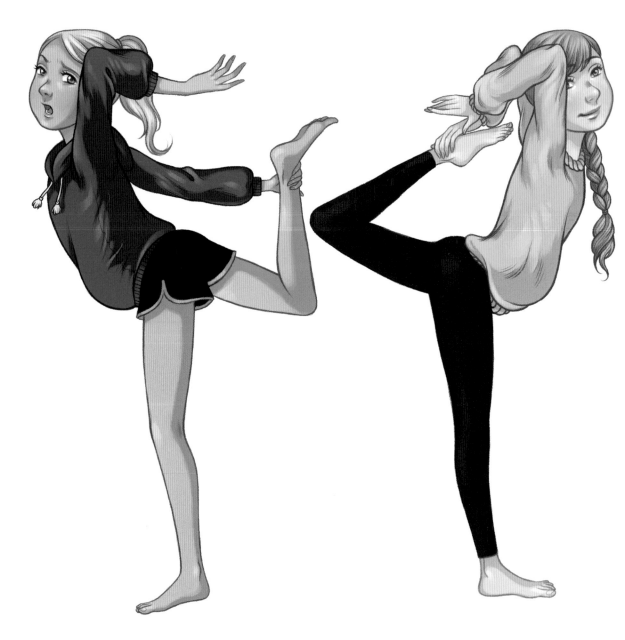

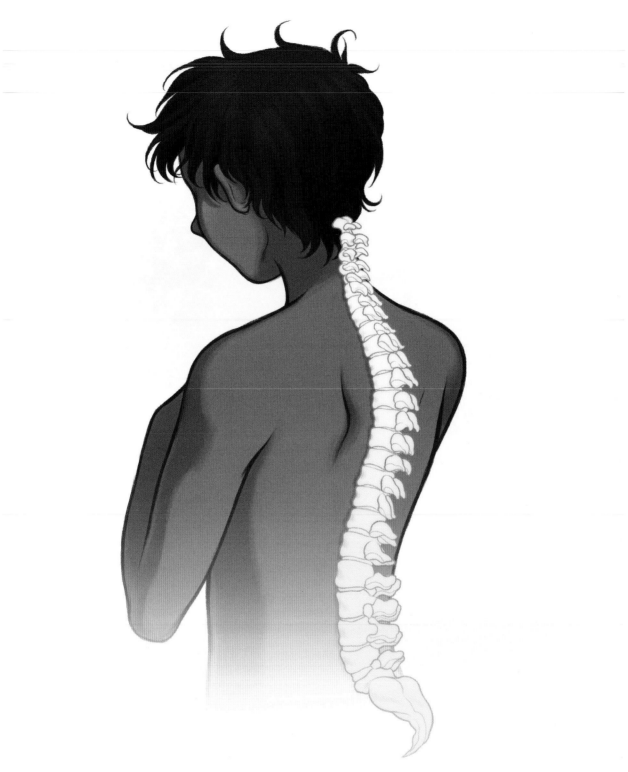

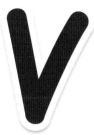 is for Vertebrae

Vertebrae are bones that make up your spine.
Yoga keeps our spines flexible and healthy.
(Do you know how many bones are in your spine?)

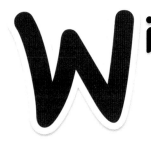# W is for Wheel Pose

1. Lay down on your back.
2. Place the soles of your feet on your mat with your heels touching your behind.
3. Place your palms underneath your shoulders.
4. Inhale and straighten your arms and legs, lifting your pelvic area towards the sky.
5. Exhale and hold the pose. Take a moment to be calm.

(Can you curve your body to look like the top of a wheel?)

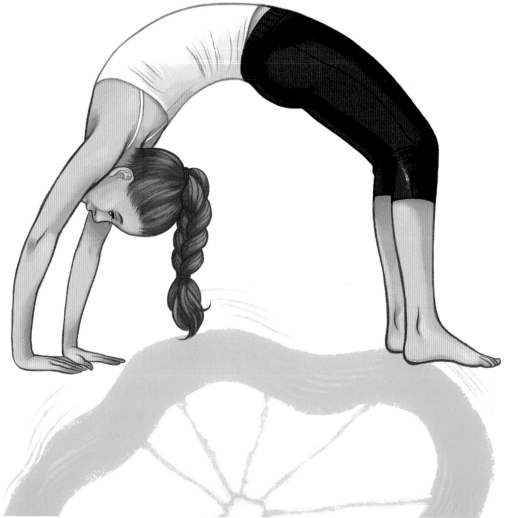

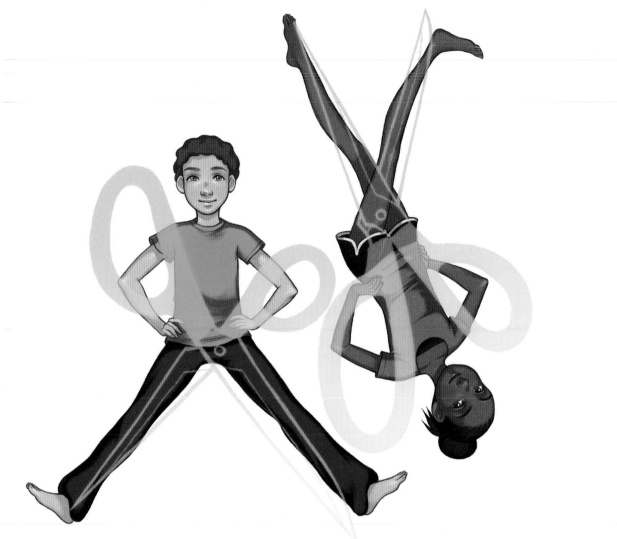

X is for making an "X" with your legs

1. Lie down on your back and place your arms at your sides.
2. Spread your legs out as far as you can.
3. Bring your legs together and criss-cross them until they look like an X.
5. Inhale and exhale as you are crossing and uncrossing your legs.

(Can you pretend you're a giant pair of scissors cutting a piece of paper?)

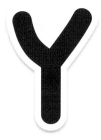 **is for Yoga**

Yoga is an ancient type of exercise. Yoga started in India a long time ago. Yoga is actually a way of life. It is all about breathing and stretching your body. Yoga helps your body connect with your mind. After practicing Yoga you will feel energetic and have a more positive outlook on life.

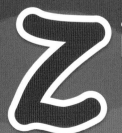

Z is for...Zzzzzzz

Yoga will allow you to sleep soundly at night. When you sleep well, you can function better in every aspect of your life.

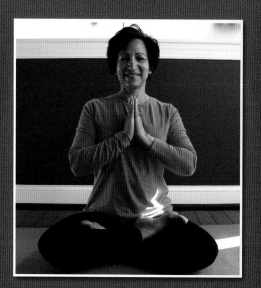

Namaskar / Namaste!

I feel extremely happy to share my book with parents, teachers and students.

I am not a certified Yoga instructor. I am sharing my experiences as a school teacher. Children these days are part of too many activities and are introduced to too many unnecessary gadgets at a very young age. I strongly feel that Yoga helps them focus and calms them. When I was a teacher, I introduced Yoga to my preschoolers, kindergarteners, and first graders on a regular basis. They loved it. I know for a fact that it has helped some of them calm themselves and be more focused. I strongly believe that children can concentrate better with practice and Yoga gives them that practice. Yoga helps make the classroom and home atmosphere more positive and peaceful.

The most gratifying feeling was that my students enjoyed doing Yoga. They loved the turning, twisting and rolling. Many liked it so much they would ask me for more poses to try. It was such a joy to see children helping each other with their poses. Yoga did wonders for their spirit of teamwork! This is why I wanted to write this book and share my experiences with you, the readers. I hope that you enjoyed reading this book as much as I enjoyed writing it. I carefully selected the most child-friendly and well-liked poses out of hundreds of possibilities. Although this book is geared toward children, I love Yoga and would recommend it to anyone regardless of their age.

I am honored that Mr. David Rosenburg, who has been a Yoga instructor in Ann Arbor since 1993, agreed to write a foreword for this book. I hadn't seen him in twelve years and asked him to write a foreword. As you saw, he very kindly agreed to help. I can't thank him enough. Mr. Rosenburg was the guru who introduced me to Yoga twelve years ago. I was suffering from back pain at the time, but now my pain is gone. I have been practicing Yoga ever since, and it has helped me tremendously in every aspect of life.

I am still in awe of the illustrations created by Jen Mundy, and I thank her from the bottom of my heart.

I owe a big thank you to my "Yogini" daughter, Roshani, for all of her help.

If you enjoyed this book, please check out my first title, *N is for Nepal*.

If you have any questions or comments, please feel free to email me at annarboranita@gmail.com.

Om Shanti Peace

Cheers,
Anita Bhandary Adhikary

Anita Adhikary has two daughters. She lives in Ann Arbor, Michigan with her husband and their cat, Columbus.